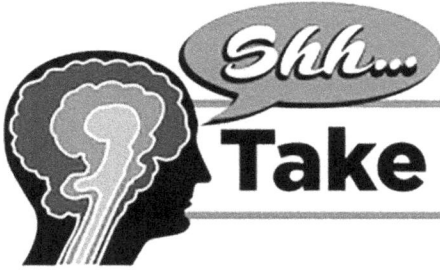

Shh...
Take A Breather®

Discover how PEOPLE OF ALL AGES CAN BECOME

*S*MARTER *H*EALTHIER *H*APPIER

SIMPLY BY CHANGING THE WAY THEY BREATHE

Shh... Shh... Shh...

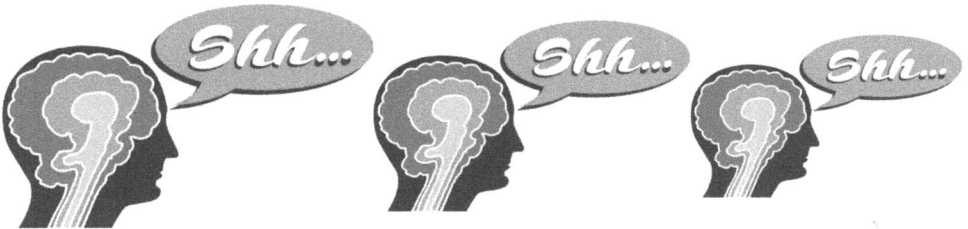

Far from being ordinary,
breathing is a transforming potential
(Carl Stough)

JANINE C. FLETCHER

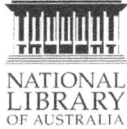

A catalogue record for this book is available from the National Library of Australia

NATIONAL
LIBRARY
OF AUSTRALIA

Publisher:
ASPG (Australian Self Publishing Group)
P.O. Box 159, Calwell, ACT Australia 2905
Email: publishaspg@gmail.com
http://www.inspiringpublishers.com

National Library of Australia Cataloguing-in-Publication entry

Author: Fletcher, Janine C.

Title: **Take A Breather**/Janine C. Fletcher

ISBN: 978-1-922618-67-2 (pbk)
ISBN: 978-1-922618-99-3 (eBook)

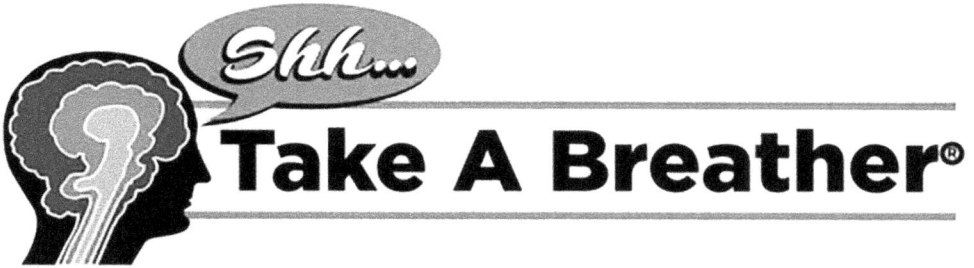

Shh... Take A Breather®

Discover how PEOPLE OF ALL AGES CAN BECOME
*S*MARTER *H*EALTHIER *H*APPIER
SIMPLY BY CHANGING THE WAY THEY BREATHE

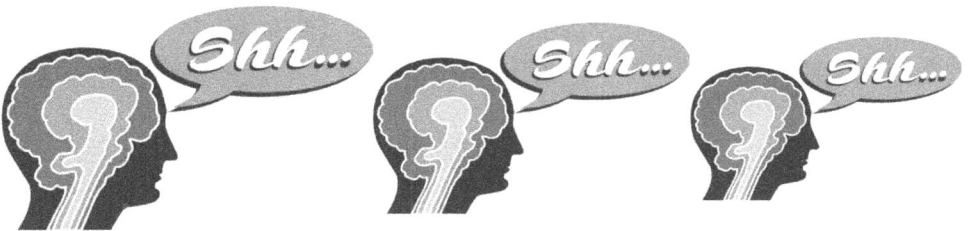

*It may be hard to believe,
but 9 out of 10 adults breathe incorrectly,
thereby impairing their health and
exacerbating anxiety and depression.*

(Dr Joseph Mercola)

DISCLAIMER

The suggestions in this book for personal growth are not meant to substitute for the advice of a trained professional such as a medical doctor, psychologist, therapist etc. It is the individual's responsibility to consult such a professional in the case of any physical or mental symptoms.

Table of Contents

Chapter One
THE
ONE THING

have a question for you.

What's the one thing that you're doing right now, and every minute of every day, that is either having a negative or a positive effect on you?

This **one thing, <u>depending on how you're doing it,</u>** will either be:

- Causing you to be in a negative frame of mind

  OR

  in a positive frame of mind

- Making you feel anxious, angry, defensive, agitated

  OR

  making you feel calm, peaceful, relaxed, friendly

- Triggering your body's stress response

  OR

  activating your body's natural healing ability

- Having a negative impact on your training, sports performance and recovery time

  OR

  having a positive impact on your training, sports performance and recovery time

- Helping you to focus, concentrate, learn easily, and be productive

  OR

  making it difficult for you to focus, concentrate, learn, and be productive

- Enabling you to access your creativity

  OR

  causing you to be 'stuck' for ideas

- Causing you to be defensive, irrational, reactive, and impulsive

OR

improving your ability to respond in a calm, rational way and make conscious choices

- Increasing

OR

decreasing your pain levels

If the impact this **one thing** is having on you **depends on how you're doing it,** then it stands to reason that if you learn how to do this one thing in such a way that it is having a positive rather than a negative impact, you will have more control over

- your frame of mind, how you feel and the choices you make;
- your anxiety and stress levels;
- your health and your pain level;
- your learning ability, your creativity, concentration, and productivity;
- your sports performance and recovery time;
- how you respond to others and even how you feel about yourself.

That's quite a significant impact this **one thing** can have on your life**.**

Take a few minutes to ponder...

Which would you prefer to experience?

Positive frame of mind	Negative frame of mind
Relaxed, peaceful, friendly	Anxious, angry, defensive
Body's natural healing ability	Stress response

Improved performance and faster recovery time	Poor performance and long recovery time
Concentration, focus, being productive, and ease of learning	Difficulty with concentration, focus, productivity, and learning
Creativity and inspiration	Stuck for ideas and struggling
Respond in a calm, rational way and make conscious choices	Defensive, reactive, impulsive, irrational
Decreased pain level	Increased pain level

What do you think this **one thing** could be?

Chapter Two
IT'S BREATHING!!

*Breath is the very essence of life and drives
all the other functions of the body.*

*We can't do without breathing,
but we can do it badly for a long time.*

*Poor or dysfunctional breathing in turn leads to a
whole host of other problems, including poor digestion
and bowel function, decreased ability to control pain,
poor posture, stress, depression, migraine, poor
sleep patterns, lack of concentration and so on.*

*The whole act of breathing in and out
creates a lymphatic movement, and poor
breathing and posture will also contribute
significantly to lymphatic congestion...*
(Julian Baker, *Bowen Unravelled*)

Breathing is the most important act in life.
(Carl Stough)

Maybe you were expecting something a little more complicated. The impact your breathing pattern (simply the way you are breathing) can have on you mentally, physically, emotionally, and spiritually is certainly very significant; but because it is so simple, practical and basic, its powerful effects are often overlooked.

Many people are unaware of just how great an influence their breathing pattern could be having on all aspects of their lives.

...how little was known of the potentials of breathing and how desperately people needed to know about the influence of breathing upon health and wellbeing...
(Carl Stough)

As an educator, I am really passionate about sharing this information. This book truly could change your life.

My purpose in writing this book is to

- make you aware;
- give you the opportunity to experience for yourself the astounding side-effects of changing your breathing pattern, and
- share some of my research with you

Becoming aware

Reflect on the following ...

When we are born, breathing is the first thing we do to signal that we're alive ... and what we stop doing to signal that we are no longer alive—it's the first and the last thing we do.

I wonder just how significant that is.

*To breathe is to be alive. Could
breathing hold a key to life?*

*What is the connection to the way we breathe
and the way we are experiencing life?*

We can do without food and water for days and still survive, but we can only do without breathing for a matter of minutes.

To thrive every cell in our bodies needs an abundant supply of oxygen.

When we are stressed or anxious it becomes difficult to breathe.

When we are happy, calm and relaxed, it is easy to breathe.

On average a person may take between 17,000 to 30,000 breaths a day.

Become aware of how you are breathing right now ...

... is it relaxed, soft, slow, gentle, deep, easy? Or laboured, heavy, shallow, fast?

Where in your body do you feel the air going? Into your throat, chest or belly?

Does it feel comfortable or uncomfortable for you?

How are you feeling... physically...mentally... emotionally... spiritually?

An opportunity to experience for yourself the astounding side-effects of changing your breathing pattern...

I'm going to guide you through three different breathing patterns. I encourage you to follow the instructions and do them for yourself, so that you can get a sense of the phenomenal impact simply changing the way you are breathing can have.

1. The first one is **a shallow, rapid, chest breathing pattern.**
   Place one hand on your chest. Take around ten short, shallow, fast breaths. Feel the movement of your chest and probably also your shoulders.

   - Notice what breathing like this is doing to you
   - How is it making you feel?
     (more than likely breathing like this is beginning to make you feel very uncomfortable, anxious, annoyed, angry, defensive...)

2. The second breathing pattern is **a slow, gentle, deep, abdominal breathing pattern.**
   Place one hand on your tummy. Take around ten slow, gentle, deep breaths. Feel the movement of your tummy—expanding as you breathe in, and contracting again as you breathe out.

- Notice what breathing like this is doing to you
- How is it making you feel?
  (more than likely breathing like this is beginning to make you feel more comfortable and much better than the previous breathing pattern)

3. The third breathing pattern is called **Take A Breather** or the **solar plexus breathing pattern.**

   This breathing pattern is similar to the above abdominal breathing pattern but is has three unique features.

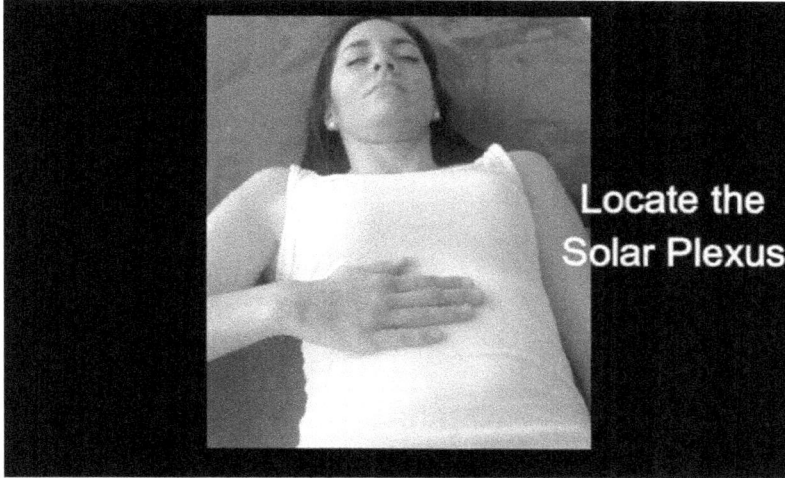
Locate the Solar Plexus

1. The focus is on expanding the muscles and rib cage, to create the space for your lungs to fill to their full capacity, and the outward movement of the solar plexus area.

2. There is a significant pause between the inhale and exhale.

3. The exhale is very slow.

Interestingly, the **Take A Breather** breathing pattern mimics the natural movement, expansion and rhythm we experience when we yawn.

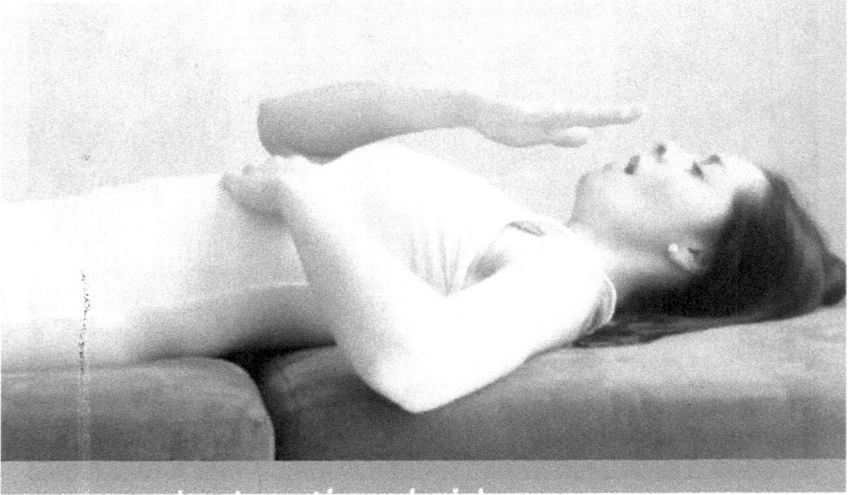

To experience this for yourself, place your hand in front of your mouth, open your mouth wide and take in some air ... this should make you yawn.

As you yawn pay particular attention to

- The expansion of your rib cage and muscles
- The outward movement of your solar plexus area
- The significant pause between the inhale and the exhale
- The slow exhale

NB. I have noticed that there are some people who have difficulty yawning. If you are one of those people, please keep reading as I know some strategies and techniques that may assist you.

Another way to experience this movement is to pretend you are smoking a cigarette

As you pretend to smoke a cigarette, pay particular attention to

- The expansion of your rib cage and muscles
- The outward movement of your solar plexus area

- The significant pause between the inhale and the exhale
- The slow exhale

This same movement is also experienced when we take a breath when we are laughing or crying.

Now that you're familiar with the movement, expansion and rhythm ...

Let's **Take A Breather**

Chapter Three
LET'S TAKE
A BREATHER

To experience *Take A Breather* or the solar plexus breathing pattern, simply repeat these 4 steps:

1. Take a slow, gentle, deep breath in through your nose.

2. Feel the outward movement of your solar plexus area as you expand your ribcage, chest and abdominal muscles.

3. Pause; gently keeping your muscles in that expanded state. Never hold your breath, just pause.

4. Very slowly breathe out.

When you're familiar with the four steps, close your eyes and continue to *Take A Breather.*

(If you're not sure if you're doing the technique correctly, or you would prefer to listen to a guided audio when you *Take A Breather*, I suggest you purchase the ***Take A Breather*** app).

On the app there is an instructional video, two guided audios (one is approximately five minutes and is more suited to children, and the other is approximately ten minutes and is more suited to adults). It also has other suggestions if you need extra assistance, as well as additional information, activities and processes.

The single most important thing
You can do to improve a child's health
is to establish nasal breathing.

(Dr John Flutter)

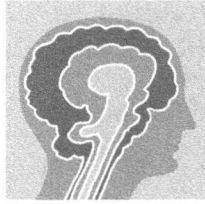

available from the App Store for $9.99

https://appsto.re/au/szB5_.i
https://play.google.com/store/apps/details?id=au.com.
janinefletcher.takeabreather

After five or ten minutes, notice how you feel ...

What changes have you experienced after Taking A Breather?

It might be interesting to write these changes down so you can refer back to them as you learn more.

After Taking A Breather I feel ...

Some of the common responses from children and adults the first time they experience the *Take A Breather* breathing technique are things like:

I feel calm, relaxed, comfortable, safe, confident, stronger, smarter, more gentle, soft, peaceful

I feel like I could do anything

It's refreshing

It makes me feel happy inside

It makes me feel more alive

I feel less stressed

It makes my worries go away

I feel ready to learn

It helps me to not be angry

I feel like nothing in the world can hurt me

I feel like I just filled up with joy

It lifts a heavy weight off my shoulders

I have a more positive perspective

It brings out the best in me

It's such a relief

They're pretty impressive outcomes, don't you think? And they are achieved after just after a couple of minutes of *Taking A Breather.*

If there was a pill you could take to get results like these (without any nasty side-effects), people would be lining up to buy it.

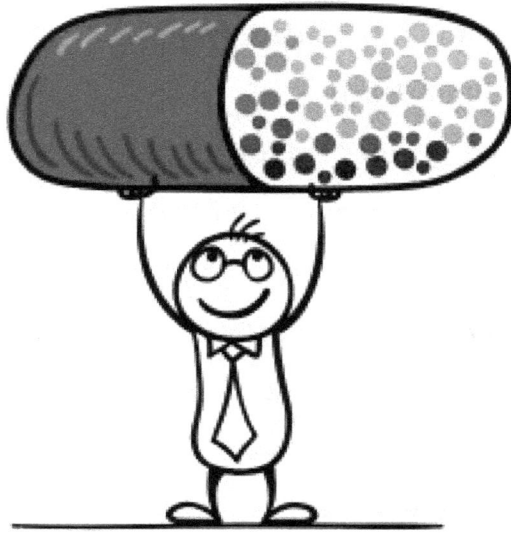

MAGIC PILL

The following information from Dr Frank Lawlis helps to explain what is happening inside the brain and body to produce these kinds of responses.

There are over 2,000 organs and hormones that can be affected positively or negatively in a matter of minutes by shifting your breathing pattern.

*Taking quick, shallow breaths usually signals to the brain that a threat exists, which stimulates the **stress response** and therefore establishes destructive thinking patterns.*

Conversely, taking slow, deep breaths, usually signals to the brain that the coast is clear, and all is well.
*(Retraining the Brain, **2008 Dr Frank Lawlis**)*

The **stress response** Dr Lawlis is talking about is often called the 'fight-or-flight' response, and sometimes also the 'freeze-or-flop' response. This is our in-built survival mechanism and affects the body in such a way that anything that isn't necessary for survival—things like thinking, learning, digestion—shut down. This is a very handy response if you're in a life threatening situation; but for most of us, on a daily basis, this survival response can be triggered by psychological threats and fears.

We can trigger the **stress response** by worrying about things. Either things that have happened in the past or things that may happen in the future, fear of saying the wrong thing, fear of not being liked, fear of making a mistake, financial concerns, general anxiety, feeling overwhelmed, feeling like you need to protect yourself, being defensive ... anything like that.

Your physical life isn't actually in danger—it just feels like it is.

Even negative self-talk, whether it is directed towards yourself or someone else, is enough to trigger a **stress response.**

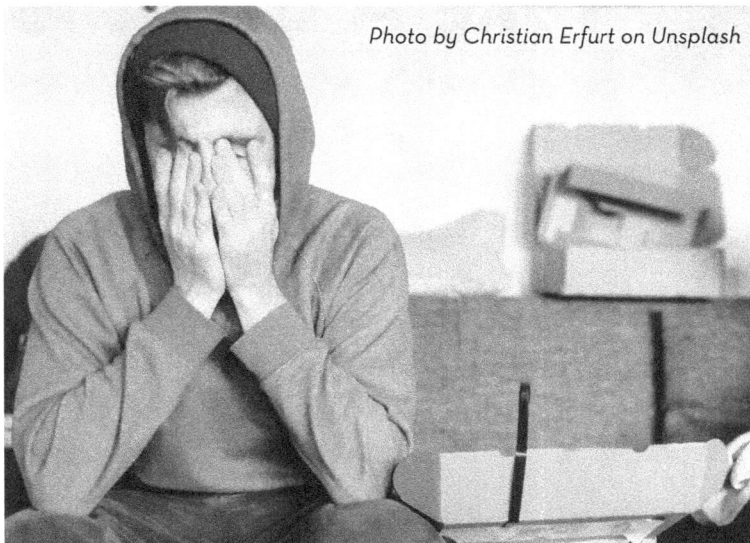

Photo by Christian Erfurt on Unsplash

When we consider improving our lives,
we often overlook our breathing habits.

(Anders Olsen)

The good news is that of all the physiological responses to stress, **breathing is the one we can consciously control.**

This means that we can have so much more personal power in our lives and that we can benefit greatly by consciously controlling our breathing.

Using my research data, I've categorised the benefits of *Taking A Breather* into three major categories, covering mind, body and spirit. You'll find them under the headings of **S**marter, **H**ealthier and **H**appier (SHH)—kind of a cool match for *Take A Breather*—SHH ... *Take A Breather*.

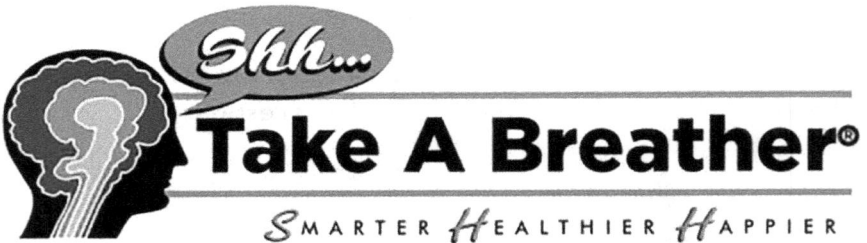

GOOD NEWS

The good news is that of all the physiological responses to stress, **breathing is the one we can consciously control.**

Chapter Four

TAKING A BREATHER CAN MAKE YOU SMARTER

You've probably already experienced this for yourself. When you're stressed, you can't think clearly or concentrate, and you're certainly not in a receptive learning state.

The stress response is our survival mechanism, so when we're stressed, functions that are not necessary for survival (like thinking and learning) shut down.

The triune brain model is a theory of the functioning of the human brain by Neuroscientist, Dr Paul D. MacLean (National Institute of Mental Health, Washington). While the triune brain model is somewhat outdated and simplistic, I think it helps to stimulate thinking about the different aspects of being human and how these relate to life, learning and behaviour.

The triune brain model suggests that the brain is made up of three distinct areas.

The Triune Brain

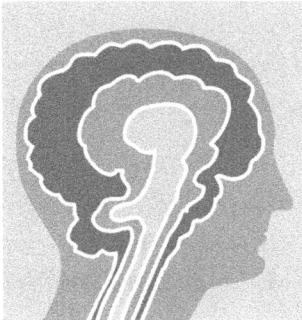

■ **Neocortex** responsible for "higher" brain functions

■ **Limbic System** or mid-brain responsible for emotions and memory

■ **The Reptilian Brain or Survival Brain** responsible for base drives

Neocortex

- Is the seat of academic learning
- Is the intellectual and creative brain
- Contains approximately 70% of the brains ten billion neurons
- Has the ability to exhibit healthy integration of emotion and rational thought in response to stress
- Is the most effective mode for rational thinking
- Is the centre for all intellectual and abstract thought
- Is capable of innovation and a high-level of creativity
- Is actively involved in discrimination and focusing abilities are strong
- Loves challenges, change and possibilities

Limbic System

- Processes emotions
- Important to memory and learning
- Immune and **autonomic nervous systems** are regulated in this area

The Autonomic Nervous system – controls the internal environment. It governs breathing, heart rate, digestion and other physiological activities such as physical responses to emotion (i.e. sweating palms) that often accompany fear.

There are two divisions of the **Autonomic Nervous System**: The **Sympathetic Nervous System** (also Known as the 'fight or flight' system and the **The Parasympathetic Nervous System** (also known as the 'rest and digest' system).

The impact on the body's internal environment depends on which system is being activated.

For example, if the **Parasympathetic Nervous System** (PNS/ Rest and Digest) is activated, breathing will be slow, gentle, and

---

deep, heart rate will lower, digestion will take place, and access will be available to the functions of the neocortex.

Neocortex and PNS

Positive frame of mind	
Relaxed, peaceful, friendly	
Body's natural healing ability	
Improved performance and faster recovery time	
Concentration, focus, being productive and ease of learning	
Creativity and inspiration	
Calm, rational responses and ability to make conscious choices.	
Decreased pain level	

If on the other hand the **Sympathetic Nervous System** (SNS/ Fight or Flight) is activated, breathing will become more rapid and shallow; heart rate will increase, digestive function will decrease, and a person will operate from the survival/reptilian brain.

The Reptilian Brain -Survival Brain

- The main responsibility of this brain is to ensure survival and to maintain routine bodily functions (breathing, heartbeat, etc)
- It is also responsible for:
  - ✧ monitoring the outer world through sensory input and then activates the body to physically respond in ways that ensure survival
  - ✧ Controlling of self-preservation

- ✧ Automatic responses to stimulus
- ✧ Safety and physical survival
- It is unable to reason
- Has no innovation or sense of risk-taking

Under stress, extra electrical activity and blood supply are needed in the survival areas of the brain (**the reptilian and limbic system**). They are directed away from the **neocortex** where understanding and high-level thought processes can occur.

... the reptilian (survival) brain is the part of the brain that takes over when we encounter danger or stress because it initiates and regulates the body's fight-or-flight response.
The reptilian brain oversees the mind/body's survival, ensuring that basic needs are met before other, higher functions can proceed smoothly.
(Carla Hannaford, Ph.D., Neurophysiologist)

Survival and SNS

	Negative frame of mind
	Anxious, angry, defensive
	Stress response
	Poor performance and long recovery time
	Difficulty with concentration, focus, productivity and learning
	Stuck for ideas and struggling
	Defensive, reactive, impulsive, irrational Increase pain level

Only one of these systems operates at any given time...

As we learned in the previous chapter,
we can consciously control our breathing.

This means we can have some control
over which system we activate.

If we breathe slowly, deeply, and consciously, we will calm the SNS and survival brain and activate the PNS, allowing access to the neocortex.

Some of my research ...

Taking A Breather overrides the stress response and makes us **S**marter because it:

- Improves your concentration and ability to focus
- Allows you to be in a receptive learning state
- Activates the neocortex of the brain enabling you to be capable of innovation, high level creativity and problem-solving ability
- Improves academic performance and is key to overcoming learning difficulties
- Enables effective rational thinking and your ability to make conscious choices - to respond rather than react
- Promotes a 'growth' mindset - loving challenges, change and possibilities

I'm sure you can imagine the potential benefits of such a simple tool as *Take A Breather* to help students to be able to focus and concentrate, calm, relaxed classrooms, students being in a receptive learning state and able to access their creativity.

What I observed when I was assessing the students' breathing patterns was that those students who were experiencing learning difficulties, were anxious or had behaviour problems, were often classic 'chest breathers'.

In July 2012, after 11 years of research, I first introduced *Take A Breather* to a Primary School in Geelong, Victoria. I assessed the breathing patterns of nearly 500 students and then taught them the *Take A Breather* breathing technique.

My observations merely supported the research I'd done on how the brain manifests 'chest breathing' and the 'stress response'. But it was intriguing just the same. I began to wonder if simply changing a child's breathing pattern would help that child to overcome his/her learning difficulties.

In July 2013, I attended a seminar by Dr Grant Sinnamon, a neuroscientist from Queensland, who has developed the REPAIR Model. As I listened to Dr Sinnamon's presentation on brain development, the different functions each area of the brain is involved in, and the difficulties deficits in particular areas cause, I started thinking that perhaps 'breathing' would help to improve brain function and restore these deficits.

> *Without the brainstem (reptilian brain) functioning at an optimal level, we are automatically going to have problems with higher order functions.*
> **Dr Grant Sinnamon**

I had the opportunity to speak with Dr Sinnamon and he said he also believed that 'breathing' was a key factor in improving brain function. In the early days of *Take a Breather*, I had several professional discussions with Dr Sinnamon. We would share our ideas and experiences, and he would explain the sometimes intricate science behind what at first seemed like miracles to me.

The first of these occurred when I was listening to a Year 3 boy ('A') read.

The words 'A' was saying didn't match the words in the book. He was making up a great story, but it wasn't what was written on the page. I asked 'A' if his solar plexus area felt open or closed. (I have discovered that this is an indicator of stress or impaired function). 'Oh, it's closed,' he replied. As we had learned that *Taking A Breather* was meant to improve brain function, I suggested 'A' go and Take a Breather until his solar plexus area felt open.

To my surprise, when 'A' returned to read to me, he read perfectly—no mistakes, and exactly the words that were written on the page!

After a few more experiences like this, I was inspired to develop a simple 3-step process using *Take A Breather* to target specific areas. By that I mean:

- Whatever it is you want to improve, focus on or do that activity first
- Then *Take A Breather* for a few minutes or until your solar plexus area feels open, and you feel calm and relaxed
- After you've *Taken A Breather*, simply repeat the same activity and notice what changes have taken place

Some other examples:

A 15-year-old reads well but is unable to remember most of what he has read. He *Takes A Breather* for a few minutes and is now able to recall most of what he reads.

A Year 4 girl can't think of what to write about and is stuck for ideas. She *Takes A Breather* for a few minutes and comes up with a great idea and is excited to continue writing.

A Year 5 boy who reads fluently but doesn't understand what he is reading, scores 3/10 for a comprehension test. He *Takes A Breather* for a few minutes and scores 9/10 for the same test.

A Year 5 boy who reads quite well but is unable to recall what he has read, or answer comprehension questions, says he finds reading boring. He *Takes A Breather* for a few minutes and when he continues reading, he begins to laugh. The book he is reading is suddenly funny and he now understands what he reads. He is also able to answer comprehension questions.

These are just a few examples of the incredible impact *Taking A Breather* for a few minutes has had on students.

Does it always work this quickly?

In my experience so far, I'd say often, but not always.

I'll share with you another example where it took a bit longer, and if you're a teacher, it may just give you a different perspective on those students who seem to take forever to do their work.

'T' was in Year 5 and was taking forever to complete his work. His task was to copy some information from another book. The threat of having to complete his work at recess caused an emotional plea from 'T'.

'But I can't help it. I can't go any faster!' he said.

I asked 'T' to explain to me what was happening.

He explained that when he looked at what he needed to copy, by the time he went to write it, he had forgotten what the words were.

I said it sounded like something wasn't quite connecting in his brain and suggested that he *Take A Breather*.

I checked on 'T' a few minutes later but he was still struggling. I suggested he *Take A Breather* for a bit longer.

When I checked again, there was still no change. 'T' did *Take A Breather* for the third time... the bell went. 'T' still hadn't completed his work, but he went out to recess anyway.

I was a bit disheartened because I had expected instant results.

The next day "T' was asked to complete a similar task. After a little while 'T' came to me and said, "I don't know what happened, but I can do it now!"

My desire to be able to offer *Take A Breather* to any student who may be struggling was the main reason I was prompted to create the *Take A Breather* app.

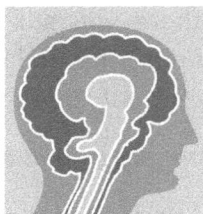

Take A Breather app – available from the App Store for $9.99

https://appsto.re/au/szB5_.i
https://play.google.com/store/apps/details?id=au.com.
janinefletcher.takeabreather

The app has been designed in such a way that you will know all that you need to know to use *Take A Breather* for yourself.

On the App you will find:

- An instructional video,
- Additional activities for those who need extra assistance
- A 5-minute guided audio (more suited to children)
- A 10-minute guided audio, (more suited to adults)
- and Seven simple 3-step processes:

    1. To improve reading
    2. To reduce stress, anxiety, worry
    3. For creative ideas/solutions
    4. To ease headache/pain
    5. To feel better
    6. To improve eyesight
    7. To address individual needs

If you are wondering if *Take A Breather* will help either your child, yourself, or anyone else, just notice the breathing pattern. Any time a person is struggling in a particular area, chances are the breathing pattern is shallow—chest breathing ... or they may not be breathing at all! So, Taking A Breather would help.

I often suggest parents and teachers become familiar with the Take A Breather breathing technique and processes on the app before they guide a child through *Taking A Breather*. This way they will be able to match the instructions at a pace that suits the child, and be able to watch for any changes in breathing pattern.

It is such an honour and a privilege to be able to facilitate some of these changes and so heartwarming to see some of the transformations that can take place.

I'd like to share one more example with you. This one was a little more involved and a more long-term project.

One day I was approached by 'A''s mum. 'A' was in Year 4 and was just not making any progress in maths. 'A''s mum knew of my background and asked if I could suggest what she could do to help 'A'.

I told her that I'd seen some promising results from using *Take A Breather* and offered to work with 'A' once a week at lunchtime.

'A' had received extra tuition and support all through school and at home in maths. Her reading was very good, but her maths showed little or no progress. In Year 4, 'A' even struggled to count in twos.

Each week I worked with 'A', we focused on a different mathematical skill or concept, and 'A' would reinforce this at home by first *Taking A Breather* (allowing her to be in a receptive learning state), before practising the skill or concept.

Three years later, I contacted 'A' and her mum to ask her to write a testimonial about her experience with *Take A Breather*. *This is what she said:*

When my daughter, 'A' was in Year 4, I was really concerned because she still wasn't making any progress in Maths. No matter how often we practiced or how much extra support she had, she struggled to remember even the most basic number concepts. From the time she started school, anything to do with numbers and Mathematical processes just didn't 'click' with her.

After just 6 weeks of working with Janine and using the Take A Breather breathing technique to target Maths deficits, 'A' was able to learn more, retain more and had the confidence to do more, than she had in nearly 5 years at school.

'A' is now in year 7 and her lack of progress with Maths is a thing of the past. Her recent comment that 'I enjoy Maths', speaks volumes. She continues to learn and develop her understanding of number and Mathematical concepts. Maths doesn't scare her anymore; - she has the confidence to 'have a go' as well as the ability to work Mathematically, (her Maths brain is working!); - she 'gets it' now.

I don't guarantee that *Take A Breather* will be the single answer to all of a child's learning difficulties, but I'm pretty sure it will help. The very least it will do is allow your child to be in a receptive learning state.

I can't begin to imagine what it's like for a child to have to front up to school day after day, year after year, and struggle to learn; - just not 'getting it', not understanding why, thinking that there is something wrong with them.

If simply *Taking A Breather* can help even a little bit, it's worth doing and if it fixes the problem altogether, then that's brilliant.

As you may have guessed, my background is mainly in primary teaching and education. I have also trained as a masseuse, Bowen therapist and kinesiologist. With regard to *Take a Breather*, education is the area in which I've had the most experience. However, there would be similarities in the workplace especially as far as the ability to focus, concentrate, be productive, stress manage-ment and health and wellbeing are concerned.

Regular *Take A Breather* breaks in any workplace would definitely be beneficial.

TESTIMONIALS:

'M' Age 8

'M' experiences learning difficulties with mathematics and has difficulty recalling the simplest equations from time to time. She is also a nervous child and eager to please, so it was causing her great anxiety in the classroom.

We saw an immediate response during the session and her teacher has reported a noticeable improvement in the last few months. Janine's experience as a teacher together with her breathing technique has definitely helped M – she now has the tools to enable her to focus on problem-solving and manage the way she reacts when she gets stuck.

(M's mum)

'A' Age 7

'A' is doing very well with her reading and also concentrating more on her maths. Thank you very much for the Take A Breather technique. We can see that it is helping her in a big way. She does not rush and is a lot calmer with her schoolwork.

(A's mum)

We've now covered how *Taking A Breather* can make you **S**marter. How *Taking A Breather* can make you **H**ealthier is what we'll look at in the next chapter.

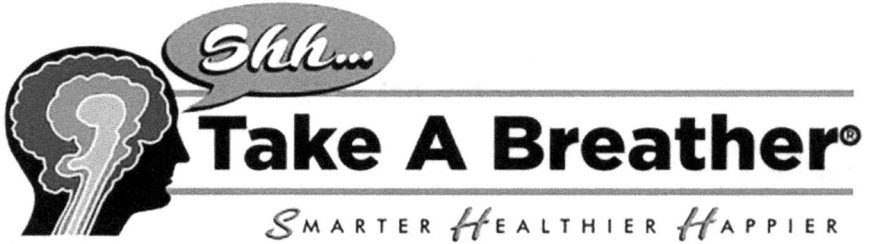

Chapter Five

TAKING A BREATHER CAN MAKE YOU HEALTHIER

A quick Google search will tell you that 75-90% of doctors' visits are due to stress-related illnesses. To consider breathing as a part of any wellness and healthcare plan is definitely a good idea, and it is supported by science as well as common sense.

The insidious effects of constantly elevated stress hormones include memory and attention problems, irritability, and sleep disorders.

They also contribute to many long-term health issues, depending on which body system is most vulnerable in a particular individual.
Bessel Van Der Kolk (MD)

Slow, deep breathing supports the body's ability to heal naturally, engages the Parasympathetic Nervous System (the Rest and Restore Nervous System) which helps to digest stress hormones.

Stress hormones lead to cellular inflammation which is the root cause of all degenerative disease.
(Christiane Northrup MD)

So, on the one hand we have the stress hormones produced by the fight or flight (survival) response, and on the other hand we have a way of engaging the rest and restore or Parasympathetic Nervous System, which helps to digest stress hormones.

If we don't have a way to balance the stress response with the rest and restore response, we can become exhausted and unwell.

Mental health and anxiety are also areas where considering breathing as part of the healthcare plan is definitely a good idea.

---

*By sitting and mindfully breathing for ten minutes a day,
in as little as eight weeks you can strengthen
the part of the pre-frontal cortex involved in
generating positive feelings and diminish
the part that generates negative ones*
Richard Davidson, Ph.D.

I came across some other interesting ideas in this area in a book called *The Master Key System* written by Charles F. Hannel (1866-1949) ...

... the breathing apparatus responds to every thought

*... when you are 'tired' or 'discouraged', your body
is starved by short, irregular breathing supply*

*... A person cannot breathe slowly and deeply
and be sad, fearful, critical or judgemental*

*A depressed person is not in the
habit of breathing deeply.*

One lady I spoke with who suffered from anxiety had been told by her doctor to take some deep breaths. She'd also seen it recommended in magazines and on health programs, but no one had actually shown her how to breathe in a way that helped—until she learned the *Take A Breather* technique.

If someone is suffering from anxiety, they're usually in the habit of 'chest breathing'. Telling a 'chest breather' to take deep breaths can actually make them feel worse, unless they change where they are breathing from. I have found that learning the *Take A Breather* breathing technique is really beneficial for people suffering with anxiety.

I also found when teaching *Take A Breather* to a group of young, teenage men who had been diagnosed with anxiety, that just understanding what was happening on a physiological and neurological level when they experienced anxiety, gave them a sense of relief and empowerment.

Another area where *Take A Breather* can be beneficial is training and sports performance.

A little while ago I was sent an article from a fitness magazine titled, 'Breathe Better. Train Better.' In the fitness industry, the importance of effective and efficient breathing is obvious.

Because *Take A Breather* activates the Parasympathetic Nervous System (rest and digest or rest and restore), it also helps with recovery time.

In summary

Some of my research

Taking A Breather makes us **H**ealthier because it

- Reduces stress and anxiety, and has a positive impact on stress-related illnesses

- Supports the body to heal naturally

- Engages the Parasympathetic Nervous System, the rest and restore nervous system, which helps to digest stress hormones

- Improves sports performance and aids recovery time

- Provides an abundant supply of oxygen to every cell in the body, which is essential for full functionality

- Helps to reduce pain levels

TESTIMONIALS:

'E' *Age* 40

For no special reason I started to suffer from anxiety at the age of 40 and the slightest issue could give me cause for concern.

'Take A Breather' provided techniques to manage my anxiety – from understanding the feeling, to managing my response.

I now use the technique when I feel anxious and also when I need to have clarity and focus on a task.

'L' *Age* 13

I use the app when I feel like I'm going to have a panic attack and also when I am feeling anxious or uptight about something. In the mornings sometimes I feel this way before school and after I use the App, I feel calmer, and my breathing isn't all frantic. The App helps me with being less stressed about something and less worked up about different things.

In the next chapter we'll look at how *Taking A Breather* can make you **H**appier.

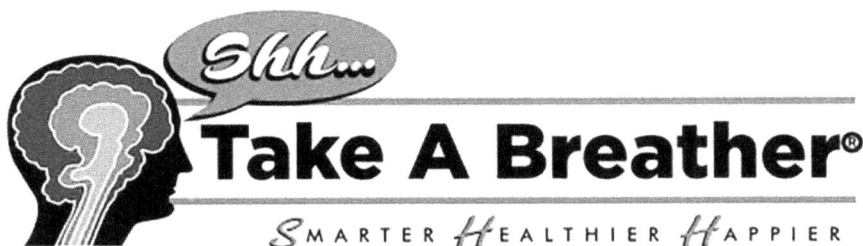
Shh... Take A Breather®
SMARTER HEALTHIER HAPPIER

Chapter Six

TAKING A BREATHER CAN MAKE YOU HAPPIER

As breathing is the one physiological response to stress we can consciously control, by *Taking A Breather*, it is possible to override the stress response, calm yourself down and respond in a more rational, wise and constructive manner. The sooner you are able to do this, the easier it will be.

When you become aware of the first signs of a stress response — tense muscles, shallow breathing, increased heartrate, a tightening in the solar plexus area — you need to stop and *Take A Breather.*

I'm not suggesting that you suppress your emotions. I've found that if there is a build-up of suppressed emotions, until that emotion is expressed, a person may actually have difficulty *Taking A Breather.*

It can be useful to think of emotions as energy. If you keep suppressing an emotion, it can build up and explode out of proportion to the situation, or be misdirected.

So-called negative emotions often have a positive message — they can be a signal that you need to make some change in your life — lifestyle, relationship, direction, being true to yourself, and so on. Sometimes, an emotion like anger for example, that is triggered by some injustice, can be a motivator to take some positive action. It's more a matter of using the energy in a **constructive, rather than a destructive, way.**

So, if you feel an emotion like anger inside, allow yourself to feel it. Just see it as energy, let it run its course, and let it go (ideally if you can do this in private, you won't be taking it out on anyone else).

Once this anger, or whatever emotion it is, is out of your system, you can *Take A Breather* and calm yourself down. When you're in a calm, relaxed state, you'll usually be able to get a different perspective on the situation and respond in a more constructive way. Basically, you'll have more control over how you respond.

On the *Take A Breather* App there is a simple 3-step process that is designed to help access our inner wisdom and get a different perspective when we are stressed, worried or anxious.

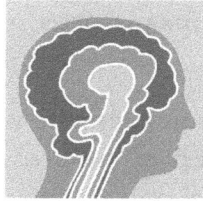

available from the App Store for $9.99

https://appsto.re/au/szB5_.i
https://play.google.com/store/apps/details?id=au.com.
janinefletcher.takeabreather

I'll tell you a story that demonstrates this beautifully. The story is about two primary school students, but I'm sure you'll be able to imagine how it might relate to people of all ages, in all types of situations.

After recess one day, a young girl was in tears and said that another girl had been mean to her. Both girls were pretty upset so I suggested they go and *Take A Breather,* and when they were feeling better, to see if they could come up with any good ideas about improving the situation.

After about five minutes, I asked each girl what they had come up with.

The 'victim' said, *'Well, I know I can be over sensitive, and I really don't have to take any notice of what someone says to me.'*

The 'bully' said, *'I know I can be pretty mean, and I really don't want to be like that anymore.'* She then apologised for her behaviour.

Taking A Breather can help us to access our innate wisdom and bring out the best in us.

Obviously, not all relationship challenges will be solved simply by *Taking A Breather*. It is certainly more effective if all parties involved do it, but it helps to be aware of just how harmful the stress response can be to our relationships and ourselves.

When we are stressed, we tend to be negative, closed minded, irrational, and defensive. Our thoughts, feelings and behaviours when we are in this state tend to be negative and destructive. When we feel safe, happy and relaxed we are much more likely to be understanding, rational, compassionate and 'at our best'.

Doing something as simple as *Taking A Breather* can make such a difference.

In the long term, the results can be even more impressive.

Remember Richard Davidson's quote from Chapter 5.

By sitting and mindfully breathing for ten minutes a day, in as little as eight weeks you can strengthen the part of the pre-frontal cortex involved in generating positive feelings and diminish the part that generates negative ones

Richard Davidson, Ph.D.

In this chapter, the focus has been on How *Taking A Breather* can make you **H**appier.

Some of my research ...

- Aids in the production of 'feel good' chemicals such as serotonin
- Helps to 'bring out the best in you'
- Promotes resilience and the ability to 'bounce back' faster from challenges
- Allows you to see things from a different perspective. Seeing things from a different perspective changes the way you think, feel and respond
- Positive emotions: peace, kindness, understanding, love, joy, compassion and gratitude come to the surface
- Gives you access to more positive, constructive and empowering thought patterns

TESTIMONIALS:

'N' (Teacher) Age 43

...Within a matter of minutes, I went from being highly stressed to very calm and peaceful. This allowed me to put my 'issues' into perspective in a positive way. The most empowering and reassuring aspect of this is that as Janine guided me through the process, I was able to maintain my privacy and make these changes within myself. Very quick, very easy, very powerful!

'J' (EEN -Nurse) Age 53

The first time I tried the Take A Breather technique, I experienced a profound shift of all mind chatter. I found myself in a peaceful and calm state of mind quite quickly. As I listened to the Take A Breather app, Janine's voice kept me there; - reminding me to stay on task. After the

10 minutes guided audio, the peaceful feeling stayed, and I had a clarity of thought which lasted for hours.

'A' (mum of two)

Take A Breather was recommended to me by a friend. I was curious as to how breathing could help my two daughters.

Life just seems so busy these days and I wanted to lessen the anxiety, mood swings and overall unhappiness I was seeing in my girls.

Janine and the Take A Breather technique have been awesome. She has given the girls the tools they need to turn many situations and their thoughts into positive ones. Learning to breathe properly enables them to think about things calmly and resolve situations well. It is a bonus to be able to do this at any time of the day. I have also reaped the benefits of Take a Breather in my hectic day to day life.

I would recommend this to anybody. It is truly amazing how breath can change things for the better.

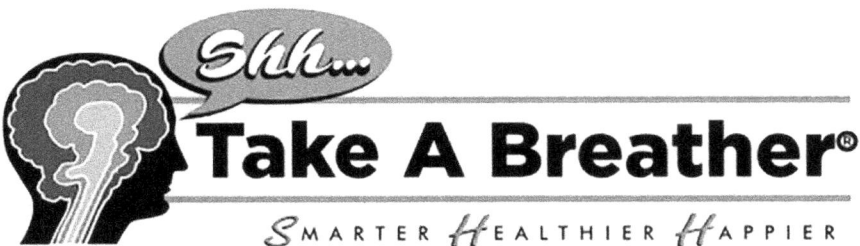

Chapter Seven
A POWERFUL TRANSFORMATION TOOL

Far from being ordinary,
Breathing is a transforming potential

(Carl Stough)

Simply changing the way you are breathing can
help you to be Smarter, Happier and Healthier

How incredible is it that most of us have grown up not knowing this?

And, what a difference it can make to our lives when we do know.

Breathing is the one thing that every single human being on the planet has in common. It's so simple, it's so powerful... and now you do know.

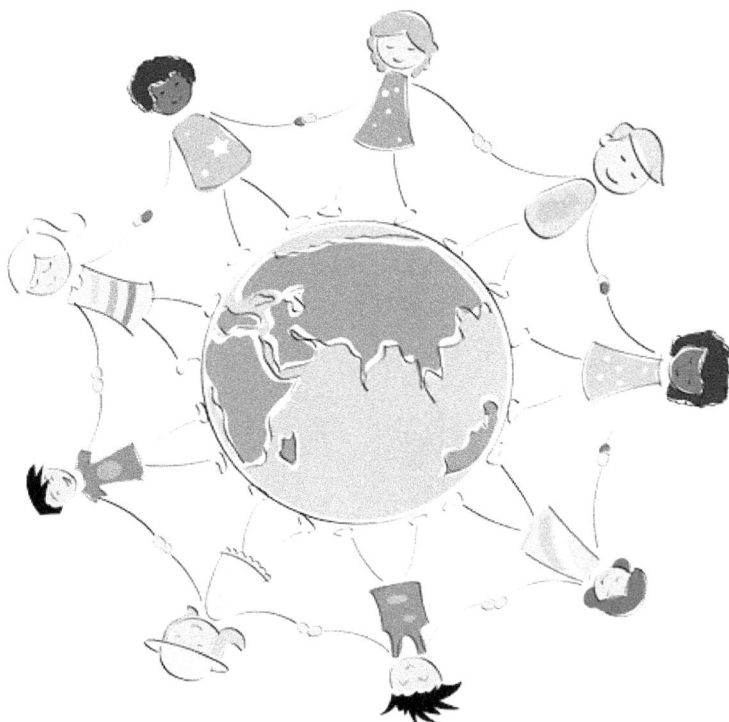

(Image from VectorJunky)

This is information that will serve you for the rest of your life, in so many ways, when you remember to use it.

I personally like the *Take A Breather* breathing pattern because it is safe, and it mimics the body's natural movement, muscle expansion and rhythm. It's also very easy to learn. I've taught it to children as young as 4 years old through to Mum is now 90 years old.

I've not practised or trialled any other breathing techniques to the extent I have *Take A Breather,* so I've only been able to tell you about my experiences with *Take A Breather.*

So far, the *Take A Breather* breathing technique has yielded some pretty impressive results and I hope you will be inspired or curious enough to use *Take A Breather* for yourself. The least that will happen is that you will give your mind, body and spirit a chance to rest and restore and, you just might experience a 'miracle' yourself.

You know enough right now to begin using *Take A Breather.*

The *Take A Breather* app will also guide you step by step in using this powerful transformation tool.

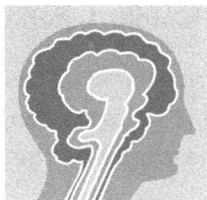

Take A Breather App – available from the App Store for $9.99

https://appsto.re/au/szB5_.i
https://play.google.com/store/apps/details?id=au.com.
janinefletcher.takeabreather

Many of my experiences with *Take A Breather* 'miracles' have been unexpected and came about just because I was curious and open minded enough to 'have a go'.

The next *Take A Breather* experience I'm going to share with you was one of those 'miracle' ones that I couldn't wait to share with my 'go-to' neuroscientist at the time, Dr Grant Sinnamon.

A few years ago, I had successfully used my kinesiology skills and vision exercises to improve my brother's blurred vision. When he got up in the morning, his vision was blurry, and he didn't want to start wearing glasses. At the time, the kinesiology and vision gym work that we did had rectified this.

Years later, I was visiting my brother in Queensland, and I noticed that he'd started wearing glasses to read small print. We were sitting in the beer garden at the Kin Kin pub in Queensland. I was returning to Victoria the next day and didn't really have much time or what I needed with me to repeat the kinesiology and vision gym treatment, so I decided to see if Taking A Breather would improve his eyesight.

Again, I just followed the simple 3-step process:

1. I gave my brother something to read.
(*He needed to hold it at arm's length, squinting and struggling to make out the words as they were blurry for him*).

2. He closed his eyes and I guided him through *Taking A Breather* for around five minutes.

3. I asked him to open his eyes and read the same thing again.
(*This time he held it just in front of him and was able to see the print clearly*).

I hadn't really expected it to work, but we were both astounded and delighted that it did. The improvement in his eyesight lasted for around three weeks before he needed to repeat the 3-step process again.

When I returned home, I went through the same process with other family members and friends, and I got similar results.

I had no idea how to explain this, so I gave neuroscientist Grant Sinnamon a call. He said it absolutely could happen and went into great detail about what would be happening neurologically for something like this to occur.

Dr Sinnamon also said that it wouldn't work for everyone — it depended on what had caused the deterioration in the first place. This has also been my experience — some people experience major improvements and others minor; and some, no improvement at all.

As a general guideline, if you do experience an improvement in your eyesight after *Taking A Breather,* you will only need to repeat the process when your eyesight becomes blurry again.

The simple 3-step process for improving eyesight can be found on the *Take A Breather* app.

The following link will take you to an interview with Chris Reed on 'The Bowen Buzz'. You will hear of Chris's personal experience of using the Take A Breather technique to improve his own eyesight.

https://www.bowenbuzz.com.au/bowen-buzz/episode-5-take-breather-janine-fletcher/episode-5-janine-fletcher/

Sometimes to make positive changes, all you will need to do is *Take A Breather*. Other times you will still need other intervention — other therapies, techniques, education or special assistance. Nevertheless, if you include *Take A Breather* as part of your intervention, anything else you do will be more effective.

The impact breathing has on our quality of life is beginning to become more widely known, and once you experience it for yourself, you will be amazed that you haven't made the connection to breathing and quality of life before. It is so obvious once you know.

Breathing is the most powerful tool that everyone has within their reach; whatever they're doing and wherever they are.

I hope I've opened your mind to the incredible possibilities offered by *Taking A Breather*. Once you learn it, you've got it for life.

I encourage you to become more aware of your breathing pattern throughout the day and take regular *Take A Breather* breaks. Follow the 3-step process for any area you struggle with or would like to improve, and take notice of the difference *Taking A Breather* is making in your life.

TESTIMONIALS:

'M' Age 41

I initially used 'Take A Breather' to improve my eyesight. I tested my eyesight before using the APP for the first time and after. I definitely noticed an improvement.

After a couple of weeks, I realised I hadn't been reaching for my reading glasses as much. When I did start reaching for them more, I 'took a breather' again and my eyesight became better. So now, every few weeks I 'Take A Breather' just to make my eyesight stronger.

I also love the way it makes me feel calmer and clearer in the head.

'J' Age 52

The Take A Breather technique is nothing short of a miracle, with life-changing results accessible by each and every one of us. It has certainly changed my life. Although I am by nature a positive type of person, there are times in my life when I have and do experience anxiety, self-doubt and being stuck in a negative headspace. It can be a horrible, debilitating place to be. It could be brought on by a job interview, work dead-line, weight gain, exhaustion or just a bad day all around. We've all had one of those days.

Since being introduced to Take A Breather I am so much more in control of all aspects of my life. After just 10 minutes of TAB, I feel lighter, thoughts are clearer and there is a calmness that brings clarity and confidence back. I encourage you to Take A Breather and see for yourself; - it's phenomenal

I've seen some amazing changes take place simply by a person *Taking A Breather* – **improvements** in reading, comprehension, maths, handwriting, sports performance, dancing, drawing, creativity, pain levels, anxiety and stress levels, attitudes, eyesight, perspective, relationships ...

I hope you too witness or experience all of these improvements and more.

Be curious, 'have a go' and see what you discover.

The potential applications of *Take A Breather* are endless ...

Further Information:

www.janinefletcher.com.au

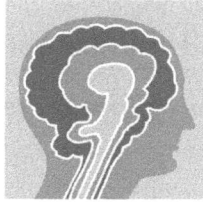

Take A Breather app available from the App Store for $9.99

https://appsto.re/au/szB5_.i
https://play.google.com/store/apps/details?id=au.com.
janinefletcher.takeabreather

This little book really could change your life. It takes less than 30 minutes to read, but what you learn will impact the rest of your life, showing you how you can have so much more personal power.

- Your frame of mind, how you feel and the choices you make
- Your anxiety and stress levels
- Your health and pain level
- Your learning ability, creativity, concentration and productivity
- Your sports performance and recovery time
- How you respond to others and even how you feel about yourself